Is Your House Making You Sick?
A Beginner's Guide to Toxic Mold

Andrea Fabry

Is Your House Making You Sick? A Beginner's Guide to Toxic Mold

ISBN-10: 1523732482
ISBN-13: 978-1523732487

Cover photo copyright © by Andrea Fabry

Edited and designed by Sherry Parmelee

Connect with Andrea via email at andrea@momsaware.org.

Visit momsAWARE's website at www.momsaware.org.

Visit Andrea's blog, "It Takes Time," at www.it-takes-time.com.

For my mother,
My dearest friend and encourager.
I miss you still.

Contents

Introduction 1

Chapter 1: First Steps 3

Chapter 2: Surface Mold 15

Chapter 3: Water Intrusion 21

Chapter 4: Mold Remediation 25

Chapter 5: Cross-Contamination 31

Chapter 6: Medical Testing 37

Chapter 7: Detoxing 41

Chapter 8: When Others Don't Understand 47

Chapter 9: Legal Recourse 53

Chapter 10: Your Next Home 59

Chapter 11: Hope After Mold 63

Appendix A: Our Family's Story 67

Appendix B: Resources 81

Notes 85

About the Author 89

Introduction

A Word from Andrea

We left our home and everything in it on October 4, 2008. Seven months later, our daughter Shannon visited the home wearing a mask and a hazmat suit. We learned the hard way that hidden water damage can wreak havoc on a family's health.

As our family attempted to navigate the road to recovery, I quickly discovered how little was known in mainstream medicine about the physical, neurological, and emotional effects of toxic mold. I took my determined mother's heart and vowed to learn everything I could about the connection between the indoor environment and human health. The more I learned, through my own research and my study in the field of Building Biology, the more passionate I became about sharing this knowledge with others. Poor building practices matter when it comes to our health. Water leaks, left unattended, have the potential to do harm

While mold is ubiquitous to our environment, not all molds are created equal. Just like members of the mushroom family, some mold species are harmless, while others are poisonous.

Not all mold situations are catastrophic. When mold is found early and properly remediated, environments can be restored and health maintained. Some people are more tolerant of the effects of mold than others. There is no one-size-fits-all when it comes to toxic mold. My hope is that this resource will give you a starting point, whatever your situation.

If you're experiencing impaired health due to a mold or other environmental issue, you're not alone. Many are suffering and most are without knowledge. Awareness is the first step—one you've already taken by picking up this book.

I hope you find help, guidance, and most of all hope from my family's experience and the knowledge I never knew we needed until that fateful day in 2008.

My thanks go out to toxicologist Dr. Jack Thrasher for caring enough to tell us what we needed to hear. Thanks as well to Sherry and Dan Parmelee for the technological and editing assistance that has taken me from my first blog to this book. To my kids, for their unwavering support and determination. And to my husband, Chris, for his enduring love.

Chapter 1

First Steps

How can I determine if I have a mold problem?

Your first step when mold is suspected is to acknowledge a connection between health and your environment. This is one of the most overlooked aspects of wellness, despite the World Health Organization's estimate that one in eight deaths globally can be attributed to air pollution—with more than half of those deaths resulting from exposure to household air pollutants.[1] Since many of us spend up to 90 percent of our time indoors, it's imperative that we remain vigilant when it comes to our indoor environments.

What is mold?

Mold is part of the kingdom of fungi, a distinct kingdom that is neither plant nor animal. Fungi are identified by a genus name and a species name. For example, *Aspergillus,* a genus, can be further classified as a species with the name *Aspergillus versicolor,* or *A. versicolor.*

Mold causes biodegradation of natural substances such as food or building materials. Problematic species of mold found in indoor environments also release mycotoxins as a means to survive and multiply. These mycotoxins are carried on the mold spores and have been implicated in numerous health issues as they are readily absorbed by the intestines, airways, and skin.

Mold can be classified as either viable or nonviable. Viable means the spores are capable of reproducing. Nonviable molds are dead spores, but because the cell walls break apart and release toxins, nonviable spores are still considered hazardous.

How does mold grow?

Mold growth occurs when conditions are favorable. These conditions include:

- **Moisture.** This can come in the form of humid air, dripping pipes, or water intrusion due to flooding. Mold will grow when the relative humidity is roughly 50 percent or higher.

- **Food.** Mold will feed on wood, paper, cotton, and leather. Drywall with its paper coating offers ideal food for mold spores. Mold can grow in dirt or dust if the conditions are right.

- **Favorable temperature.** Spores will proliferate in temperatures ranging from above freezing to below 120 degrees. Summer-like temperatures (70–90 degrees) are especially conducive to mold growth.

- **Time.** Mold growth can occur in 24–48 hours or it may take as long as 10 days, depending on the conditions.

- **Stagnant air.** Insufficient ventilation contributes to moisture buildup.

Mold is an opportunistic pathogen, which means it will take advantage of any conditions favoring its growth.

What are the symptoms of mold exposure?

Every individual responds differently to toxins related to indoor mold growth. In their paper "Mixed Mold

Mycotoxicosis: Immunological Changes in Humans Following Exposure in Water-Damaged Buildings," Dr. Jack Thrasher and Dr. Michael Gray list the following symptoms:[2]

- Excessive fatigue
- Headache
- Nasal symptoms
- Memory problems
- "Spaciness"/disorientation
- Sinus discomfort
- Coughing
- Watery eyes
- Throat discomfort
- Slurred speech
- Lightheadedness
- Dizziness
- Weakness
- Bloating
- Weak voice
- Coordination problems
- Vision changes
- Rash
- Chest tightness
- Wheezing

According to their findings, females had a greater frequency of the following symptoms:

- Excessive fatigue
- Headache
- Memory problems
- "Spaciness"/disorientation
- Slurred speech
- Lightheadedness

- Weak voice
- Spasms
- Coordination problems
- Vision changes
- Rash
- Cold intolerance
- Heat intolerance
- Chest discomfort
- Excessive thirst
- Swallowing problems
- Skin flushing
- Rapid pulse
- Palpitations
- Bruising
- Swelling ankles

It's common for one family member to exhibit symptoms while another does not. If one person is away from the environment for most of the day, it's not unusual for the individual who stays home to experience more symptoms. Survey all members of the household using this list, and take note of the less obvious symptoms like digestive problems, mood swings, and vision disturbances.

How can I test for mold?

The first test is an intuitive one. Are there signs of water damage? Is there a history of flooding or plumbing leaks? Are there health issues in the family?

If the answer is yes to any of these questions, you're on the right track. Perhaps you don't suspect mold but want to rule out the presence of something toxic in your environment. It's always wise to consider toxic mold and its related biocontaminants.

If significant health issues exist, consider leaving the environment for a period of time to see if symptoms improve. Sometimes the testing can stop here. The home may be toxic enough to consider relocating permanently. Lab testing can still be valuable, however, to determine a course of action regarding your possessions. (See Chapter 5: Cross-Contamination.) It is best not to cut into any drywall or lift any carpet until you have tested the environment, since disturbing the mold spores can make the situation much worse.

Preliminary testing can be done with a simple moisture meter obtained from a local hardware store. Place the meter's probes in the suspected wall to see if hidden moisture is present.

Thermal imaging is a new technology that peeks behind walls without disturbing spores. Personal thermal imaging devices are now offered by the company FLIR ONE, available through Amazon.com and other online sellers.

There are several options for determining the presence of mold, including those listed below.

Mold plates. Inexpensive testing kits found in hardware stores, consisting of petri dishes with a growth medium into which mold spores can settle, do not "pull" the air, and therefore provide a limited picture of your air's spore content. A toxic mold issue can easily be missed when using this product.

Dust testing. A more effective method is dust testing, including the ERMI (Environmental Relative Moldiness Index) dust test. The ERMI uses a DNA-based method for identifying 36 different species of mold. Labs offering this service include Mycometrics, EMSL Analytical, and EMLab P&K.

The ERMI analysis offered by Mycometrics costs approximately $300 plus return shipping. Another option from Mycometrics is the HERTSMI test, which tests for five species of mold and costs about half the price. Both tests use a Swiffer-type cloth to obtain the dust, and both are available for purchase through the momsAWARE Online Store.[3]

If you decide on an ERMI or HERTSMI dust sample test, keep the following principles in mind:

- The species of mold in a contaminated home will vary from room to room. If you have a specific area of concern, take the dust from that room and consider a different test for other areas of the environment.

- "Historical" dust samples should be included in the testing. Sites for these include refrigerator coils, which are a 24/7 collection site, as well as any drop-down kitchen cabinet doors or air returns for heating and air conditioning.

- If you would like an overall picture of the home, take dust from various parts of the house. This will not help you isolate the source, but will let you know what types of mold you're breathing on a daily basis.

Air testing. An air test is less optimal than a dust or tape sample. However, when taken in conjunction with dust samples, it can be a valuable tool.

Tape sampling. A tape sample can be used if the mold is visible. Check with the three labs noted above for pricing and availability.

Bulk sampling. With bulk sampling, a piece of contaminated material such as drywall or carpet is cut out, bagged, and labeled for lab testing. This method of testing is risky, as cutting the drywall or removing carpet can release spores and make the situation much worse.

Mycotoxin testing. This measures mycotoxins in your environment as opposed to identifying species of mold. Mycotoxins are emitted from genuses like *Stachybotrys*, *Aspergillus*, and *Penicillium*. The test involves a sterile gauze pad used to swipe air vents, refrigerator coils, or specific items of concern like furniture or computers. Mycotoxin testing is available through RealTime Laboratories.

Hiring a hygienist. A combination of carpet dust samples, air samples, and tape lifts can be done by a professional hygienist. If you believe litigation will be involved, it is important to hire a hygienist.

Questions to ask a hygienist before hiring:

1. **Do you believe mold is harmful?** The answer must be yes.

2. **What constitutes a "safe" level of mold?** In an air sample, mold counts should be equal to or below outdoor counts. There should be no *Stachybotrys*, not even one spore, in an indoor air count. *Stachybotrys* produces dangerous mycotoxins shown to inhibit DNA, RNA, and protein synthesis. *Stachybotrys* does not typically go airborne, which is why it would be a red flag in an air test. *Penicillium/Aspergillus* (sometimes measured in combination due to their structural similarity) should be present only at negligible levels.

3. **Can I see the report?** Do not rely on a hygienist's word. It's important to see your counts for yourself, especially when it comes to levels of *Aspergillus*.

The cost associated with mold testing is often a stumbling block, but it can save you thousands in the long run.

How do I interpret my mold test results?

A hygienist is not trained in the health effects of toxic mold. If you disagree with the hygienist's conclusion about your situation, don't disregard your uneasiness. Don't be afraid to ask questions and be your own advocate. Remember that air sampling is very limited and may miss the presence of toxic genuses of mold like *Stachybotrys* and *Chaetomium*.

If you have performed your own dust sampling, consider the following guidelines when evaluating the safety of your environment.

1. Understand that all tests have limitations.

While settled dust is one of the best ways to get a picture of the air you're breathing, there is no one test that can assess all areas of a given building. The indoor environment is a complex mixture of microbes and toxins, including:

- MVOCs (microbial volatile organic compounds): gases produced by mold that create a musty smell.

- 1,3-beta-glucans: a polysaccharide component of fungi cell walls; linked with fungal infections and sarcoidosis.

- Endotoxins: part of the outer membrane of the cell wall of Gram-negative bacteria; linked with adverse immune responses.

- Galactomannan epolysaccharides (EPS): cell wall polysaccharides readily detected in house dust of homes with reported dampness; associated with respiratory symptoms in children.

All of these have the potential to adversely impact health. While air sampling, bulk sampling, and tape lifts all have their place, ERMI dust sampling remains one of the best first choices when evaluating the health of a building in regard to water damage.

2. Consider the species of mold, not just the count.

With the ERMI test, you will see spore counts of each of the 36 species of mold. When these counts are abnormally high, it may be assumed the building has the potential to harm health. Do not discount low counts of particularly hazardous molds, however. One spore of *Stachybotrys chartarum* can indicate a serious mold situation. Species of mold that are particularly dangerous include those evaluated in the HERTSMI dust test:

- *Aspergillus penicillioides*
- *Aspergillus versicolor*
- *Chaetomium globosum*
- *Stachybotrys chartarum*
- *Wallemia sebi*

3. Use the HERTSMI scoring system.

Even if you have the ERMI report, the HERTSMI scoring chart offered at the website Surviving Mold may be helpful.[4] This point system is designed to help those previously injured by water-damaged buildings, but can also be very useful for beginners. Check your report for the five significant molds listed above and tally your results according to the chart on the following page.

HERTSMI Scoring Chart

Units are Spore E/mg.	
10 points are assigned for	
Aspergillus penicillioides	>500
Aspergillus versicolor	>500
Chaetomium globosum	>125
Stachybotrys chartarum	>125
Wallemia sebi	>2500
6 points are assigned for	
Aspergillus penicillioides	100–499
Aspergillus versicolor	100–499
Chaetomium globosum	25–124
Stachybotrys chartarum	25–124
Wallemia sebi	500–2499
4 points are assigned for	
Aspergillus penicillioides	10–99
Aspergillus versicolor	10–99
Chaetomium globosum	5–24
Stachybotrys chartarum	5–24
Wallemia sebi	100–499

Once your total points have been determined, compare with the following interpretation:

< 11   Safe
11–15   Borderline—clean and re-test
> 15   Dangerous for those with CIRS (Chronic Inflammatory Response Syndrome)[5]

Interpreting ERMI Test Results

ERMI test results from two different homes are compared on the following page.

The results in the left column show a home that has low levels of contaminants, except for the abnormally high 6800 Spore E./mg of *Epicoccum nigrum*. This species is often associated with plant sources, so the homeowner removed all house plants and cleaned the air ducts, deciding to re-test in six months.

The ERMI results in the right column show a serious mold issue with high levels of critical species, shown shaded in gray. This homeowner vacated the home, leaving everything behind due to the presence of *Stachybotrys* in combination with serious health issues.

While an ERMI dust sample is often a good first step, there is no one-size-fits-all approach to assessing the health of a building. Always remember the value of your instincts as you consider the safety of an environment. You're wise to take the issue of mold seriously, even when the issue appears to be a surface one.

ERMI Test Comparison Chart

Species Identification	Spore E./mg dust Home 1	Spore E./mg dust Home 2
Aspergillus sydowii	ND	19
Aspergillus unguis	ND	3
Aspergillus versicolor	10	17000
Aureobasidium pullulans	23	400
Chaetomium globosum	<1	<1
Cladosporium sphaerospermum	2	11
Epicoccum nigrum	6800	55
Eurotium (Asp.) amstelodami	11	1000
Paecilomyces variotii	<1	<1
Penicillium brevicompactum	1	120
Penicillium corylophilum	ND	35
Penicillium crustosum	ND	150
Penicillium purpurogenum	ND	4
Penicillium spinulosum	ND	<1
Penicillium variabile	1	9
Scopulariopsis brevicaulis/fusca	<1	<1
Scopulariopsis chartarum	<1	1700
Stachybotrys chartarum	ND	14
Trichoderma viride	<1	1
Wallemia sebi	4	2800

(ND = None Detected)

Chapter 2

Surface Mold

Is it okay to use bleach to remove mold? How can I remove surface mold safely?

Because of the nature of indoor environments, it's easy for surface mold to develop—especially in the bathroom area, where air circulation is minimized. Before addressing the surface issue, it is important to rule out the presence of a deeper problem. Sometimes surface mold is due to hidden water damage. A crack in a tile or a history of a water leak may indicate a larger problem, which may require further testing and evaluation. (See the previous chapter.)

Bleach is commonly recommended as a solution for surface mold as well as mold hidden behind walls. This is a myth, however, as chlorine bleach not only emits hazardous vapors, it also may aggravate an existing mold situation.

If you are confident that the problem is a surface one, it is best to avoid bleach. While bleach does kill bacteria and viruses, it does not kill mold. It merely takes away the color and can trigger more problems because of its toxicity.

Similarly, ammonia is very irritating to the mucous membranes, and while it may be effective on surface mold spores, it does not eradicate dead spores that contain glucans, allergenic proteins, and mycotoxins.

More About Chlorine Bleach

The ion structure of chlorine bleach prevents the chlorine from penetrating porous materials such as drywall and wood. Mold's enzyme roots grow *inside* the porous materials, rendering the bleach ineffective. The water component of bleach, however, does penetrate the drywall or wood, which can foster further mold growth.

Moreover, chlorine bleach will discolor or whiten the surface being treated, leading the building occupant to believe the problem is solved—until the mold reappears.

A study of mold growth on Douglas-fir lumber notes the ineffectiveness of bleach, concluding:

> While bleach is often recommended for remediation of surface mold on wood, our results illustrate that the treatment does not eliminate the surface microflora.[6]

Natural Alternatives to Bleach

- **Borax.** Readily available, borax is an excellent antifungal agent. Create a paste with borax and water and scrub onto the area. Rinse and dry well. This can be applied several times and may be combined with tea tree oil for added effectiveness.

- **Hydrogen peroxide.** Peroxide is an effective antimicrobial without the toxic fumes that come with the use of bleach. If using 3% hydrogen peroxide, which is the dilution found in stores, simply apply directly to the mold and scrub. Certified 35% food grade peroxide, available online, may also be used, but should be carefully diluted before applying. A third option is 10% hydrogen peroxide, also found online. It need not be diluted and offers a stronger option. Always use caution, however, as anything greater than 3% may burn the skin.

- **White vinegar.** White vinegar also has excellent antifungal properties. Consider using white vinegar in combination with either of the above. Try the borax paste and follow with several sprays of white vinegar.

- **Tea tree oil.** Tea tree oil is known for its ability to kill fungus and is safe for ingestion or application to skin and hair. You can easily make a tea tree oil spray by combining water with 5–10 drops of tea tree oil. Spray on the surface to be treated. You can also add tea tree oil to a baking soda or borax paste.

- **Grapefruit seed extract.** Derived from the seed and pulp of grapefruit, GSE has excellent antifungal properties. GSE can be added to white vinegar or combined with other solutions on this list. NutriBiotic offers a reputable product, available at health food stores and online.

- **Pumice.** Pumice bars are cheap and readily available in the cleaning aisle of many big box stores. Pumice is great for any type of cleaning, including surface mold. Scrub the area with pumice and follow with any of these treatments.

- **Baking soda.** Baking soda, or sodium bicarbonate, is an effective antifungal agent by itself or in combination with other products. Make a paste with baking soda and water and scrub. Boost the effect by making your own washing soda (sodium carbonate) by heating the baking soda at 300 degrees for 30 minutes.

- **Chitosan powder.** Chitosan is derived from the chitin component of crab, shrimp, and other crustacean shells. It has noted antifungal properties. Make a paste of chitosan powder, tea tree oil, and water for an effective surface solution. Chitosan powder can be purchased from Amazon.com and other online sellers.

- **Vodka.** Vodka is a potent antimicrobial and can be applied directly to surface mold. Fill a spray bottle and spritz it on the area. Allow it to sit for 10 minutes or so and scrub with a rag or pumice stick.

Preventative Measures

The following preventative steps can help minimize surface mold issues:

- **Monitor ventilation.** If the mold is in the bathroom, is the exhaust fan in good working order? Are family members regularly using the exhaust fan? A new exhaust fan can be an excellent investment if the current one is not working properly.

- **Wipe down the shower after each use.** Even with the best ventilation, mold can grow simply because of the moisture and lack of sunlight. It may seem overwhelming to wipe down the tile after every shower, but once family members are in the habit, the tile stays clean and dry.

Commercial Cleaning Products

There are numerous products on the market today. Before making a purchase, be sure to address the following three issues:

1. **Bleach.** Avoid bleach at all costs, for the reasons noted above. Bleach will appear as sodium hypochlorite on the label.

2. **Chemicals.** Petroleum-based chemicals are a health hazard and are best avoided when tackling a surface mold problem. Clarify with the company if you are uncertain about the listed ingredients.

3. Promises. Beware of statements like "kills all mold." While a product can help reduce or minimize a problem, generic promises on a label can be misleading.

If any ingredients are unclear, contact the company for clarification. The following products are free from bleach and chemicals and are available from Amazon.com and other online sellers.

- EC3 Mold Solution Concentrate
- Benefect Botanical Disinfectant
- Bulletproof Homebiotic Spray (for surface mold prevention)

As with any mold issue in the home, surface mold is not to be taken lightly. Consider these non-toxic solutions and avoid chlorine bleach to help maintain a safe home environment.

Chapter 3

Water Intrusion

Our basement has flooded. How can we avoid a toxic situation?

While slow water leaks are often hidden, flooding is obvious and presents an urgent situation. Whether the water intrusion is due to a burst pipe or heavy rains, the key is quick action. Mold can grow within 24–48 hours. Stop the water intrusion as soon as possible and begin the drying process immediately. If you see mold growth, consult a mold remediation company for safe removal. (See Chapter 4: Mold Remediation.)

Natural disasters that involve water can present unique health hazards, requiring extra caution during the aftermath. According to the Centers for Disease Control and Prevention (CDC) publication "Mold After a Disaster,"

> After natural disasters such as hurricanes, tornadoes, and floods, excess moisture and standing water contribute to the growth of mold in homes and other buildings. When returning to a home that has been flooded, be aware that mold may be present and may be a health risk for your family.[7]

When assessing water intrusion, it's important to note the three categories of flood water as defined by the Institute of Inspection, Cleaning, and Restoration Certification:[8]

Category 1: Clean Water.

Water that originates from a sanitary source and poses no significant risk from contact, ingestion, or inhalation.

Category 2: Gray Water.

Water has significant contamination and may pose a health hazard if contacted or consumed by humans. (Dishwasher or washing machine overflow, toilet backup without feces, and water from aquariums are in this category.)

Category 3: Black Water.

Water is heavily contaminated and can contain pathogens or toxins. Anyone who comes in contact with or consumes Category 3 water risks health impacts. (Examples include sewage; floods from sea, river or lake; and wind-driven rain from hurricanes.)

What are the pathogens that may be present in flood waters? In their "Flood-Related Cleaning" report,[9] the Environmental Protection Agency notes that flood water is often contaminated with pathogens from sewage, farm animal wastes, and wild animal populations, or that occur naturally in bodies of water. They go on to offer an excerpted list of biological agents representing the pathogens that can be found in flood water and residue, including:

Parasites:
- Giardia
- Entameba

Bacteria:
- Campylobacter
- Salmonella
- Shigella
- Norovirus

- Enterococci
- E. coli
- Legionella
- Leptospira

Viruses:

- Hepatitis A
- Rotavirus
- Adenovirus
- Enterovirus
- Parvovirus

In light of the seriousness of water damage in the indoor environment, the following guidelines may help in the aftermath.

11 Guidelines for Safe Cleanup of Water Intrusion

1. Understand that time is crucial. Mold growth can occur within 24–48 hours.

2. Record details of damage with photographs or videos.

3. Prepare for difficult decisions. Border on the side of caution.

4. Keep children and pets away from flooded areas. Those entering the site should wear protective gear such as an N95 respirator mask, gloves, and goggles.

5. Recognize mold. Look for discolored walls or ceilings. Check for foul odors. Does the area smell musty?

6. Dry out the building. Open doors and windows when possible. Use fans. See the CDC's fact sheet titled "Reentering Your Flooded Home."[10]

7. When in doubt, take it out! Discard porous items that cannot be thoroughly cleaned and dried.

8. Pay close attention to and prepare to discard the following: carpeting and carpet padding, upholstery, wallpaper, mattresses, clothing, paper, wood, and food.

9. Discard contaminated building materials including drywall, insulation, and wood flooring.

10. Thoroughly clean all hard surfaces with hot water and soap. There are varied opinions regarding the use of bleach. All agree that bleach must never be combined with ammonia as toxic fumes will be released. It is important to note that while bleach does kill bacteria and viruses, it does not kill mold; it merely takes away the color. (See the previous chapter.) Other cleaning agents include white vinegar, hydrogen peroxide, borax, tea tree oil, and liquid detergents.

11. If your ventilation system has flooded, seek professional help. Ventilation systems are a magnet for mold growth and pathogenic bacteria, and once these get into your vents, health issues can escalate quickly. Qualified remediation and air duct cleaning companies can help prevent a problem by performing immediate cleaning of ductwork and HVAC systems.

Flooding creates an urgent situation that requires awareness and vigilance. Quick action will help you avoid long-term damage to your home *and* your health.

Chapter 4

Mold Remediation

How do I safely remediate my home?

Undetected water damage in the home can lead to serious mold problems, which can in turn cause serious health issues. Sometimes mold remediation is not the best solution when the damage is systemic or the health of the occupants is severely compromised. In these cases, vacating the home may be the best option.

In other situations, the water damage is isolated enough to warrant mold remediation. But tackling the mold issue yourself can often make matters worse, as opening up a wall without proper containment can exacerbate the problem.

It can be difficult to find a qualified remediator who understands the ramifications of improper mold remediation. Be wary of remediators who make promises such as "Product X is all you need to solve your problem." Don't be afraid to ask questions before signing an agreement. Keep this list handy as you interview prospective companies.

1. **Do you consider mold to be a potential health hazard?** While remediators are not health practitioners, they should understand the toxic nature of indoor water damage. They should be aware of the term mycotoxin and know the difference between a

mold allergy and a toxic response to a poisonous substance.

2. **Do you recommend testing the environment?** Some type of testing should be done before and after to demonstrate the success or failure of the project. This testing should not be done by the remediator, as this presents a conflict of interest. Testing should not be dismissed as unnecessary by a potential remediator.

3. **Do you document your work?** Contractors should document all work with digital photos. This is especially true of work related to the removal of building materials. Digital photos should be available to the customer after the work is completed.

4. **Do you contain the area properly?** This is critical. If the contractor negates the need for containment, dismiss them immediately. Proper containment includes plastic sheeting and some protection at the entrance to the containment site to avoid cross-contamination. Negative air machines (NAMs) should be HEPA-filtered and exhausted outside.

5. **Are you insured?** Some contractors operate without any type of insurance—which may bring down their pricing, but could cost you more in the long run. Look for someone who is legitimate when it comes to their business practices.

6. **Do your workers wear protective gear?** The answer must be yes. Workers should be outfitted with proper hazmat suits, respirators, and safety glasses. Disposable shoe covers should be worn onsite, as foot traffic is a major cause of cross-contamination.

7. **How do you dispose of waste material?** Waste material should be bagged and disposed of immediately after removal. Items must not be stored

on the premises. The disposal route should be as short as possible to minimize potential breakage or leakage. Bagged items should be double-bagged to avoid cross-contamination from the first bag.

8. **Do you wrap your equipment?** Air scrubbers and HEPA vacuums are inherent to the remediation process. This equipment should be contained with fresh wrap before entering your site. Equipment like this is subject to contamination from previous jobs and could make your situation worse if precautions aren't taken.

For more specifics on mold remediation, see AerobioLogical Solutions' downloadable document "A Condensed Remediation Plan for Small Microbial Particles" at the Surviving Mold website.[11]

If a contractor dismisses your questions or demeans your concerns, it might be wise to look elsewhere. Remember, you're the expert when it comes to your health. Don't be afraid to ask hard questions. Most of all, listen to your instincts as you seek to make the wisest decision for the health and well-being of your family.

What about ozone treatment?

Many companies suggest using an ozone generator to remediate a home. While ozone serves a purpose in the upper layers of our atmosphere, it is hazardous when inhaled directly. This is why the Environmental Protection Agency uses the phrase "good up high, bad nearby" to explain the dual nature of ozone. According to the EPA,

The concentration of ozone would have to greatly exceed health standards to be effective in removing most indoor air contaminants. In the process of reacting with chemicals indoors, ozone can produce other chemicals that themselves can be irritating and corrosive.[12]

Michael A. Pinto of Wonder Makers Environmental[13] agrees with the EPA assessment, saying,

> The main issue is that too many companies want to sell ozone as a magic bullet. Although it is an aggressive oxidizer, physical removal of the mold colonies is still the primary consideration of any remediation. Killing it is not enough.
> UV lights fall in the same category. They can be an adjunct to proper remediation but never a substitute for remediation. UV lights have the added difficulty of being more effective at addressing bacteria and viruses than they are at dealing with mold colonies and spores.
> In short, real remediation, particularly for individuals who have been sensitized or sickened by a water-damaged building, involves source removal under controlled conditions, detailed cleaning of surrounding areas, and evaluation/potential cleaning of HVAC systems and contents. It is labor intensive, but the tried and true methods are tried and true because they work.

When Remediation is Not the Best Option

There are times when even the best methods of remediation may not be successful. The Bible's book of Leviticus makes it clear that if mold is still present after remediation, the home is unsafe. This is a radical approach to mold, one shared by leading toxicologist Dr. Jack Thrasher.

Dr. Thrasher, author of the article "The Biocontaminants and Complexity of Damp Indoor Spaces: More Than What Meets the Eyes," says it is best to flee a home rather than remediate when serious health issues exist and a serious infestation is involved.

I have always been skeptical regarding the successful remediation of homes and buildings contaminated with fungi and bacteria from water intrusion. Buildings and homes are complicated structures. The spores of both bacteria and fungi, as well as their by-products (fine particles less than one micron to those equal or greater than the mold spores), are present in dust.

The dust can be found in all nooks and crannies of a building, e.g. refrigerator insulation and coils, areas not normally dusted, even in carpeting that has been vacuumed, under carpeting, and in wall cavities. Finally, little attention is paid to the contaminants in buildings that result from Gram-negative and -positive bacteria.[14]

As for the implications of this for those who are genetically challenged, Dr. Thrasher says:

People who are genetically challenged would be those who are genetically susceptible to such exposures. This would involve not only HLA genes but also genetic polymorphism of detoxification pathways such as Glutathione transferases and Cytochrome P450.[15]

The bottom line, according to Dr. Thrasher, is that certain contaminants will remain after a major mold remediation. This must be factored in as you consider your course of action. Homes can often be sold "as is" with full disclosure of mold issues. You might also consider remediation with intention to sell as you seek an environment without a history of water damage. If the water damage is localized and small, remediation can be safe and successful. Always consider your health first as you evaluate your next step.

Chapter 5

Cross-Contamination

If we have mold, does it mean we will have to leave our home and all of our possessions?

Not every toxic mold situation requires drastic action. However, many times a fresh start is a good idea. Unfortunately, there is no one-size-fits-all answer to this question.

Cross-contamination is an issue due to the nature of mold, its mycotoxins, and other pathogenic microbes in a water-damaged building.

Toxicologist Dr. Jack Thrasher describes the issue of cross-contamination this way:

> The toxins produced by mold are basically free radicals, i.e. they have reactive oxygen radicals that bind to fabrics and can be released with time. Also, not only *Stachybotrys*, but other dangerous molds release fine particles as well as larger particles, e.g. spores. The fine particles (less than 1 micron) permeate fabrics and are not readily removed. In addition, the mold spores bind to fabrics and can lead to cross-contamination of the new environment.
>
> Also, do not forget the presence of potentially pathogenic bacteria. They can be aerosolized and also contaminate furnishings and clothing.[16]

It's important to emphasize the microscopic size of mold spores. According to Minnesota State University Moorhead's Environmental Health & Safety webpage regarding mold,

> Most fungal spores range from 1 to 100 microns in size with many types between 2 and 20 microns. People with good vision may see 80–100 micron particles unaided, but below that range, magnification is generally necessary. To put things in perspective, you could place over 20 million five-micron spores on a postage stamp.[17]

As for the smaller particles, a study conducted in 2005 and published in the journal *Atmospheric Environment* demonstrates that "fungal fragments" may be deeply inhaled and cause significant problems. The study focuses on fragments and spores of three different fungal species (*Aspergillus versicolor*, *Penicillium melinii*, and *Stachybotrys chartarum*). All three were aerosolized by the fungal spore source strength tester. The conclusion:

> Fungal fragments released from contaminated surfaces outnumber spores.[18]

The study further notes:

> *S. chartarum* fragments demonstrated 230–250 fold higher respiratory deposition than spores, while the number of deposited fragments and spores of *A. versicolor* were comparable.[19]

A second study published in the January 2009 edition of the *Science of the Total Environment* journal concludes:

> The present study indicates that long-term mold damage in buildings may increase the contribution of submicrometer-sized fungal fragments to the overall mold exposure. The health impact of these particles may be even greater than

that of spores, considering the strong association between numbers of fine particles and adverse health effects reported in other studies (Gold et al., 2000; Magari et al., 2001, 2002; Pekkanen et al., 2002).[20]

Clearly there is more than meets the eye with toxic mold, and you are wise to ask questions about your possessions when confronted with a mold issue.

If the issue is small, simply washing items close to the source may be all that is needed. If your health is strong and you leave a contaminated environment, cleaning your belongings may be an option. If you or your children are in poor health and must leave your environment, proceed with the utmost caution regarding your possessions.

When our family vacated our home in 2008, we were advised by Dr. Jack Thrasher and a mold specialist to treat the home as if it were on fire. We left with the clothes on our backs and quickly replaced them. I'm grateful for the advice. While we may have been able to salvage some items, the extreme approach worked well for my sanity, since we were symptomatic even after we left. Had we brought some of our belongings, I might have obsessed about cross-contamination.

When the Situation is Extreme

If symptoms are severe, and the mold problem is systemic, the best choice may be to vacate the home and purchase air mattresses, a few supplies, and fresh clothing. Make your decisions about your belongings later. Once you're settled and have established a fresh environment, you can consider them. Often the desire to bring things with you lessens with time. This often means renting a storage facility for a period of time or storing your items in a family member's garage. If you're going to the trouble of moving away from a toxic environment, don't apologize for being "extreme." You want to do this right the first time. You can always bring things in, but it's very difficult to remove problematic items once they're in a new environment. A complete break from your belongings is often the best cross-contamination "test." Once you're established in your new environment, you can bring things in one at a time to see if they are a problem.

Salvageable Items

The following materials offer the best hope for thorough cleaning:

- ceramic
- glass
- metal

Pots and pans, dinnerware, and decorative items may be considered, as well as CDs and DVDs.

Problematic Items

- **Computers.** The computer fan has the potential to spew contaminants into a clean environment. Consider using your computer outside the new environment until a replacement can be purchased.

- **Appliances.** Refrigerators, washers, and dryers harbor dust in their coils and fans and are difficult to clean. Spores and spore fragments easily attach to washing machine parts.

- **Bedding.** Mattresses, pillows, and porous fabrics are difficult to clean. Since sleep plays a major role in recovery, any items associated with it are best avoided.

- **Books and papers.** While these items are among the most needed or may hold the most sentimental value, both are extremely porous and virtually impossible to clean. Store them loosely in plastic bins until a decision can be made at a later date.

- **Air purifiers.** Even if an air purifier is relatively new, it likely harbors contaminants from your previous environment—even when the filter is changed.

- **Upholstered furniture.** The stuffing in upholstered furniture is virtually impossible to clean thoroughly.

When cleaning an item for transfer to a new environment, the key is to eliminate the dust that carries the history of the home. This may be accomplished by rinsing or vacuuming. Be sure to use a vacuum with a HEPA (High Efficiency Particulate Air or High Efficiency Particulate Arrestance) filter.

Potential Cleaning Methods

The following cleaning methods may be considered, but are not guaranteed to be effective. These suggestions are based on feedback from others who have survived toxic mold exposures.

- **Ozone box.** These can be found online and properly contain the ozone. Place the item in the box and leave it overnight.

- **Sunlight.** Some have found success by leaving items outside in direct sunlight for several hours or several days.

- **Ionic jewelry cleaner.** Ionic cleaners operate by generating ultrasonic waves to remove contaminants and may be effective for eyeglasses, jewelry, and other non-porous items.

A Note About Pets

Pets are more like family members than possessions, but it's important to keep in mind that our animals have the potential to cross-contaminate a new environment. When a situation is extreme, it may be best to board them elsewhere until things settle. If you decide to bring pets with you, be sure to wash them thoroughly and shave them if possible. Pay particular attention to paws. When purchasing a shampoo, look for ketoconazole, a potent antifungal, on the list of ingredients.

Regardless of the extent of your mold situation, it is always wise to proceed with caution when it comes to your possessions. Just as we respect lightning, icy roads, and hurricanes, it makes sense to respect microscopic contaminants that can wreak havoc with our health.

Chapter 6

Medical Testing

What kind of medical testing can be done to determine if mold is doing us harm?

Medical testing for toxic mold exposure is a complex issue. Physicians are not commonly trained in the area of environmental illness, and many patients are unsure how to proceed. Sometimes your intuition is the best test. If your home has a mold problem and there are health issues in the family, you can trust the two are related. Simply remediating or leaving the home may be enough to recover your health.

Often it is better to test your environment before investing money into medical testing. However, every situation is unique. Don't hesitate to become your own health advocate.

How to Find a Doctor

The American Academy of Environmental Medicine offers a list of doctors who may or may not be familiar with toxic mold. Other organizations with an interest in environmental health include the American Board of Environmental Medicine and the Institute for Functional Medicine.

The following websites offer lists of certified mold specialists:

- Truth About Mold
- Surviving Mold

(See Appendix B for a full listing of these medical resources, including web addresses and contact information.)

Alternative medical practitioners may not specialize in illnesses stemming from mold or water-damaged buildings, but they often have a good understanding of toxicity and detoxification.

Options for Medical Testing

The following options are given as a foundation for research, rather than an endorsement of any specific test.

1. Vision Testing

The Visual Contrast Sensitivity (VCS) test measures the ability to perceive contrast in images. Patterns and shapes are presented in decreasing contrast and the individual's contrast perception is measured. A positive test indicates any number of health conditions including biotoxin exposure (a biotoxin is a poisonous substance released by a living organism such as mold).

VCS testing is not diagnostic for any specific condition, but may indicate a health problem that warrants further attention. Online VCS testing is available at the following websites:

- VCSTest.com
- Surviving Mold[21]

2. Mycotoxin Urine Testing

RealTime Laboratories in Texas offers testing designed to detect mycotoxins in the human body. Negative health effects are often experienced by occupants of water-damaged buildings due to the presence of these mold-produced toxins. RealTime offers urine tests for the following three mycotoxins:

- **Aflatoxins.** Produced by *Aspergillus flavus* and *Aspergillus parasiticus.*

- **Ochratoxin A.** Produced by *Aspergillus ochraceus* and *Penicillium verrucosum.*

- **Trichothecenes.** Produced by *Stachybotrys* and *Fusarium.*

If your doctor agrees, he or she will contact RealTime to order. You may also order these tests yourself through the Direct Laboratory Services website.[22] Look for the aflatoxin, ochratoxin, and trichothecene tests under the Allergy Testing category.

It is important to note that it may be advisable to wait until the body has begun detoxing to determine if these mycotoxins are present in the urine in higher than normal amounts.

3. **Lab Testing**

If you have a primary doctor willing to consider mold exposure as a cause of illness, ask for any or all of the following labs, which may indicate an ongoing inflammatory response to an environmental trigger like toxic mold and its related contaminants.

- **C4a.** An inflammatory marker proving to be a significant indicator of exposure to water-damaged buildings.

- **VEGF.** Vascular endothelial growth factor, a substance that stimulates new blood vessel formation and is often low in those exposed to toxic mold.

- **MSH.** Melanocyte-stimulating hormone, a critical part of the immune system and often low in those injured by mold.

- **Leptin.** A hormone that plays a crucial role in appetite and weight control, and often high in those exposed to biotoxins.

You may also ask for the full set of labs. A downloadable Physician's Order Sheet is available at the Surviving Mold website.[23]

4. **Genetic Testing**

A staggering 24 percent of the population is genetically wired to have a tough time ridding themselves of the deadly microbes associated with water-damaged buildings. For this group of individuals, the invading pathogens are not "tagged" and cleared by the body. Instead they run freely, leaving the body to deal with the attackers in any way it can—which leads to inflammation, often at the root of chronic conditions.

The genetic test is an HLA (Human Leukocyte Antigens) blood test available through LabCorp and can be ordered by any physician. Interpreting the test results is complicated, but may be facilitated by means of the Rosetta Stone, a system developed by Dr. Ritchie Shoemaker that offers a summary of the various susceptible genetic types and directions for interpretation. See Appendix B for a reproduction of this helpful interpretive tool.

As you consider these options, remember that it's vital to evaluate your home environment if there are health problems. (See Chapter 1: First Steps.) Despite the lack of knowledge in the medical community, don't be afraid to advocate for yourself. You are on the right track when it comes to making the critical connection between wellness and indoor air quality.

Chapter 7

Detoxing

How do I recover from a toxic mold exposure?

Genetics, circumstances, and individual physical makeup all play a role in determining how a person will recover from injury resulting from a water-damaged building. The following is an overview designed to stimulate further research rather than suggest a particular protocol.

Drug Options

Cholestyramine (CSM). CSM is the most commonly prescribed drug for mold exposure. CSM is a bile acid sequestrant, which binds bile in the gastrointestinal tract to prevent its reabsorption. It also works as a mycotoxin binding agent. CSM can be compounded to contain no sugar.

It is important to take CSM two hours before or after any nutritional supplements, as it will bind these as well.

Welchol is a similar binding agent and may be prescribed instead of CSM.

Antifungal drugs. These include the polyenes, the triazoles, and imidazoles, allylamines, and more. Nystatin is one example. Antifungal drugs may be prescribed in nasal spray form.

Low-dose naltrexone (LDN). Naltrexone is a medication typically used for the management of alcohol and opioid dependence. Given in low doses, it has also been proven effective in treating immunologically related disorders.

Natural Options

Often integrated with conventional medical therapies, natural options may include the various treatments and therapies listed below.

Potential Binding Agents

- Guggul resin
- Chlorella
- Activated charcoal
- Bentonite clay
- Zeolite (water is often used in the mining process, so be sure to choose a mold-free version)

Antifungals

- Garlic
- Oil of oregano
- Pau d'arco
- Olive leaf extract
- Caprylic acid (found in coconuts)
- Barberry
- Grapefruit seed extract

Glutathione Therapy

Glutathione is the body's master antioxidant and is often depleted when exposed to environmental toxins. Since glutathione is not easily absorbed when taken orally, there are options such as glutathione suppositories, patches, and nebulizing formulas. Coffee enemas have also been shown to stimulate production of glutathione, due to the palmitates found in organic coffee.

Diet as Treatment

Radical dietary change can play a major role when recovering from environmental illness. An antifungal diet is often recommended to starve the fungus, thereby halting the adverse microbial cycle that often occurs. Sugars and processed carbohydrates feed the fungus. According to natural health expert Dr. Joseph Mercola,

> This is not new information. Low sugar diets have been popularized in the battle against Candida overgrowth (Anti-yeast diet, Candida Diet, etc.), and mold thrives in similar conditions as yeast. It makes perfect sense that people with fungal infections begin to regain their health when they begin taking away the fungus' food supply.[24]

There is a great deal of confusion regarding the foods permitted on an antifungal diet. As you explore your options, remember the common avoidance points:

- Sugar
- Processed food
- Grains (with the exception of grain-like seeds such as quinoa or buckwheat)

The following diets may prove helpful to those seeking to recover from environmental illness:

- Phase One Antifungal Diet
- Bee's Healing Diet
- GAPS Diet
- Paleo Diet and/or Autoimmune Paleo Diet (AIP)
- Body Ecology Diet
- Low FODMAP Diet

Brain Retraining

The entire body is impacted by mold exposure. Digestive tracts are hit hard, and so are endocrine systems. The brain is invariably involved as well.

Brain retraining programs often play a part in recovery based on the premise that the amygdala, a critical structure of the brain, is involved with protective mechanisms related to chemical and immunological threats. The amygdala often becomes hyperreactive to environmental triggers in response to toxic exposure, without the affected person realizing it.

Examples of brain retraining programs include:

- Gupta Amygdala Retraining Programme
- Dynamic Neural Retraining System

Alternative Health Options

A wide variety of alternative health options exist. Practitioners may not be familiar with the specifics of mold exposure but can usually address the need to detox.

The numerous options available include chiropractic care, energy medicine, acupuncture, IV therapies, chelation therapies, far-infrared saunas, ionic foot baths, and much, much more.

Hyperbaric oxygen treatment has been shown to improve the brain function of mold-exposed individuals.[25]

Induced sweating through exercise and/or sauna offers unique benefits, according to Dr. Janette Hope. In her paper "A Review of the Mechanism of Injury and Treatment Approaches for Illness Resulting from Exposure to Water-Damaged Buildings, Mold, and Mycotoxins," Dr. Hope notes,

> Induced sweating will likely reduce the total overall body burden of toxins and support recovery in persons made ill from exposure to water-damaged buildings.[26]

Electromagnetic Radiation Awareness

Heightened exposure to electromagnetic fields (EMFs) can impede the recovery process and exacerbate symptoms. If you have developed chemical sensitivity as the result of an environmental trigger like toxic mold, you may find that you are also more sensitive to EMFs. These non-ionizing radiation fields have been shown to activate the synthesis of stress proteins. According to Dr. Martin Blank, author of "Health Risk of Electromagnetic Fields: Research on the Stress Response,"

> The stress response is a natural defense mechanism activated by molecular damage caused by environmental forces. The response involves activation of DNA, i.e., stimulating stress genes as well as genes that sense and repair damage to DNA and proteins.[27]

Dr. Blank notes that DNA damage (e.g. strand breaks) occurs at levels well below current safety limits. These safety standards also don't take into account our cumulative and constant exposures.

With this in mind, consider reducing your use of wireless radiation in the form of cell phones and Wi-Fi. If possible, hardwire your computer and return to a landline for phone communication. Pay particular attention to nighttime exposures and keep all devices away from your body. Turn off all routers at night or when not in use.

Important Notes

A healing crisis can occur as the detox from mold exposure begins. This is known as a Herx Reaction, an increase in the symptoms caused by toxic circulation and inflammation. It is, therefore, not unusual to get worse before getting better.

Nursing mothers need to exercise caution when detoxing. Consult with a qualified medical professional and remember that less can be more when it comes to detox. If you have left a mold environment, you have already begun treatment. It's easy to feel a sense of urgency when sorting through the various options. Mold avoidance is an excellent step.

If you are overwhelmed as you consider all of these options, remember that the detoxification process takes time. Begin with mold avoidance and diet as you consider the next step on your journey to recovery.

Chapter 8

When Others Don't Understand

What if my spouse, friend, or family member thinks I'm crazy for thinking mold can make people sick?

Because environmental health issues are not well understood among the medical community and the population at large, it's often a lonely road when trying to address a toxic mold issue. You may feel dismissed for thinking health can be negatively impacted by mold. On top of this, you may be experiencing neurological difficulties such as mood disturbances and brain fog. You begin to think you're crazy, and the lack of understanding from loved ones compounds the problem.

Be assured you're not foolish for thinking there is a connection between a water-damaged building and your health. Your job is to trust your instincts and keep moving forward despite the negative voices that suggest otherwise. Remember that you're doing the best you can in the midst of difficult circumstances.

Toxicity and the Brain

One of the best tools for explaining the connection between environment and health is found in the book *Why Isn't My Brain Working?* by Dr. Datis Kharrazian. In it he devotes an entire chapter to the subject of toxicity and the brain.

Dr. Kharrazian attributes modern-day inflammatory illnesses to such factors as diet, pesticides, chemicals in cleaning products, chemical emissions, and much more. (He mentions toxic mold in a previous book, but one can easily infer that mold is also an issue, considering the pathogenic nature of water-damaged buildings.) Dr. Kharrazian asks the question you may be asking: "Why are most people living relatively ordinary lives with all of these exposures, while others are not?" After all, everyone must have some measure of internal toxicity. The author calls it Toxicant-Induced Loss of Tolerance, or TILT. When a person suffers from TILT they aren't necessarily sick from the toxicants; they are suffering from *reacting* to them.

For people with loss of chemical tolerance, trivial exposures can trigger a long list of conditions, including asthma, migraines, depression, fibromyalgia, fatigue, Gulf War syndrome, brain fog, memory loss, incontinence, neurological dysfunction, rashes and so on. These people increasingly isolate themselves from the world and other people. They can't tolerate many indoor places, other people's scented body products, or clothes laundered in scented detergents. Even the smell of dryer sheets coming from a neighbor's dryer vent during a walk makes them sick. It's common for them to feel increasingly angry at other people and understandably so. When a scented product triggers a migraine, incontinence or symptoms of multiple sclerosis, the person wearing it can seem cruel and selfish.[28]

What triggers this extreme level of reactivity? The author lists four possible causes:

- Poor glutathione activity (everyday levels of a compound can only trigger an immune problem if glutathione is depleted)

- Breakdown of immune barriers (lungs, gut, and blood-brain barrier)

- Poor T-cell function (immune cells that regulate and balance the immune system)

- Chronic inflammation (symptoms include bloating, skin rashes or eruptions, joint pain, brain fog, depression, anxiety, chronic pain, chronic fatigue, and autoimmune flare-ups)

While the issues surrounding this loss of environmental tolerance are complex, Dr. Kharrazian's explanation offers a bit of sanity to those who are perplexed by the growing number of individuals suffering from environmentally-induced illness.

Given the lack of awareness surrounding the issue of environmental illness, it's easy to see why toxic mold exposure is often divisive and isolating. Keep listening to your gut and educating yourself and others as best you can.

Toxic Mold and Marriage

Dr. Lisa Nagy has a passion to educate doctors and medical professionals in the area of environmental medicine. Dr. Nagy became severely ill following a toxic exposure in her home. Trained in the field of emergency medicine, she searched long and hard to find help and hope. In her article "Household Mold and Marital Discord," Dr. Nagy emphasizes the role of genetics and accumulated environmental exposures when looking at an individual's health and susceptibility to disease.

> My personal experience and research have led me to believe that mold and mycotoxins at home or work (followed by pesticides and other chemicals) are the most unrecognized environmental exposures today.[29]

Dr. Nagy notes that environmental illnesses occur four times more often in women than men, and often women are deemed to be crazy when in truth they are toxic.

The mental changes are related to: a lack of oxygen to the brain from inflamed vessels due to the poison they have absorbed, high adrenaline and low cortisol, a severely damaged autonomic nervous system and direct toxicity from whatever toxin is the cause (such as mold, mercury or toluene).

When a male-female couple has been exposed to toxigenic mold, pesticides from tenting or spraying, or other chemicals such as formaldehyde in new kitchen cabinets, women often experience symptoms first and often different symptoms than men. They have classic chemical sensitivity symptoms: "I am exhausted, depressed and sometimes frantic. But my husband does not find perfume, air fresheners and the detergent aisle of the grocery store offensive. Yet he is mean and belligerent, is losing his memory, his balance and has skin problems, but people think he is fine and that I am the fruitcake." For this they often separate.[30]

Dr. Nagy cites a 1998 study that showed a negative impact on the adrenal health of female rats exposed to trichothecene, the mycotoxin emitted from various species of mold including *Stachybotrys*. When the females or neutered males were given testosterone, adrenal damage was prevented. According to Dr. Nagy, this illustrates why men with ten-fold higher levels of testosterone than women have less incidence of fatigue, stress intolerance, allergy, inflammation, and chemical sensitivity.

If you're reading this chapter because someone you know is struggling with a hyperreactive immune system and you're wondering if mold can really be that bad, my suggestion is to embrace them despite your skepticism. Honor any requests they may have. If they need you to change your clothes to be around them, tell them it's okay. If they ask you to refrain from wearing perfume, oblige them. Let them know you're behind them. Cheer them on. A word of reassurance and acceptance can do wonders for their health.

If you're the one feeling alone and misunderstood—keep going. Don't wait for onlookers to say the right thing or to understand. Continue to educate yourself and remain confident as you navigate a difficult and often lonely road.

Chapter 9

Legal Recourse

Where can I find legal help?

Because of the confusion surrounding the issue of toxic mold, it is difficult to obtain knowledgeable and reliable legal assistance. As yet, there is no official federal "mold law," which creates obstacles when trying to recoup losses. This is changing, however, as awareness grows.

When evaluating a course of action, it is always wise to count the costs before proceeding. Legal action can be costly not only in terms of your finances, but it can also impede your recovery due to the added stress. However, there have been numerous successful lawsuits ranging from disability claims to tenant rights to damages awarded for improper mold remediation.

Who to sue?

If you have been injured by toxic mold, your first step is to identify the party or parties that may be liable. This of course depends on whether you own or rent, or whether the injury occurred in a public building such as a school or workplace.

When You Own

According to the consumer-friendly website Nolo.com, if you own the building, the following parties may be liable depending on the circumstance. (There is no need to choose;

you can include all parties who may be responsible for the mold issue.)

1. **Homeowners' insurance.** In most cases, your first stop should be your homeowners' insurance policy. Whether your policy covers your type of mold infestation will depend on what the policy says. You'll need to carefully read the policy to find out what it covers and what it specifically excludes from coverage.

   - **Perils covered.** Coverage may specifically include certain types of "peril," meaning specific bad events such as a fire or a roof leak. If the cause of your mold infestation is a covered peril, you may be in luck. For example, if the cause of the mold infestation is a leaky roof, and roof leaks are one of the perils listed in your policy, then the insurance company is probably obligated to cover the cost of mold remediation.

   - **Exclusions.** Most homeowners' policies also have a list of "exclusions," meaning bad things that are not covered by the policy. These typically include things like termite damage or mold infestations that develop over time.

   In dealing with your insurer, you have at least one ace in your hand. Insurance companies are bound by a legal doctrine called the "covenant of good faith and fair dealing," meaning that, in dealing with a policy-holder, the insurance company is held to a heightened standard of conduct.

   In practical terms, this means that if your insurance company drags its feet, tries to trick you or wriggle out of the terms of your homeowners' policy, or otherwise plays fast and loose with you, you may have an additional legal claim against it for violation of the covenant of good faith and fair dealing.

2. **Builder or contractor.** If the mold infestation is the result of shoddy construction or materials or a failure to install proper ventilation, you may have a legal claim against the builder, general contractor, or one or more subcontractors for negligence (the failure to be reasonably careful). Some states require builders or contractors to guarantee their work in the form of a warranty; you may be able to claim that the builder or contractor violated or "breached" such a warranty.

3. **Architect or engineer.** If the mold infestation is the result of poor architecture or engineering, such as a failure to include proper ventilation in the design of the home, you may have a claim against the architect or structural engineer for negligence. Some states require architects or engineers to guarantee their work in the form of a warranty; you may also be able to claim that the architect or engineer breached that warranty.

4. **Construction supplier.** If you can show that the mold infestation in your home was "imported" into it by way of moldy construction materials such as siding or drywall, you may have a claim against the commercial supplier of the mold-infested materials.

5. **Prior owner.** Most states require the seller of a home to disclose any known problems such as the presence of a mold infestation. If the prior owner knew of the presence of mold but did not tell you when you bought your home, the owner may be liable to you for violating these disclosure laws.

6. **Realtor.** The seller's realtor (who is an agent of the seller) may also be liable for selling you a home with a mold infestation.

7. **Property inspector.** If you hired a property inspector to inspect your home before you bought it, the inspection company may be liable to you if it missed a mold infestation. You will need to carefully review the property report you were given, especially the language at the beginning regarding the scope of the inspection and any disclaimers.

8. **Condominium association.** Because of the special status of owners in a condominium complex, the condo association may be on the hook for a mold infestation, especially if it occurs in a common area.[31]

When You Rent

Under the landlord-tenant laws of most states, landlords are subject to a legal doctrine called the "implied warranty of habitability," which makes the landlord responsible for keeping the rental property free of health hazards such as a mold infestation.

Because the implied warranty of habitability is an obligation imposed by state law—whether the landlord likes it or not—it overrides any language in your lease that is inconsistent with that responsibility. So be skeptical and persistent if your landlord denies responsibility for a mold infestation under the terms of your lease.

If your landlord is dragging his or her feet, you may be able to get action by contacting your local housing authority. If you are seeking compensation for an injury or damage to your personal property, however, you will likely need to take legal action.[32]

Can I sue a mold remediator?

Sometimes a mold situation is aggravated by poor mold remediation. Again, due to the lack of federal standards, it is difficult to pursue legal action against a remediator. However, some states do have certification and remediation laws. The following is adapted from The Policy Surveillance Program, a visionary project designed to provide information about laws and policies that influence the public's health.

As of January 1, 2016, the following eleven states have mold remediation statutes:

- Florida
- Illinois
- Kentucky
- Louisiana
- Maine
- Maryland
- New Hampshire
- New York
- Oklahoma
- Tennessee
- Texas

Four states have laws that establish civil penalties for failure to comply with mold laws: Kentucky, Louisiana, New York, and Texas.

Florida, Louisiana, and New Hampshire are the only three states that have laws or will have laws that establish criminal penalties for failure to comply with mold laws.

Only Texas requires photographic evidence to prove that the mold remediation was properly conducted.

Four states require that mold workers receive training in proper procedure for mold remediation: Louisiana, New York, Tennessee, and Texas.

Three states require third-party verification that the mold remediation was done properly: New York, Oklahoma, and Texas.

Eight states have laws or will have laws requiring certification (rather than just training) of individuals and enterprises engaged in mold remediation services: Florida, Illinois, Louisiana, Maryland, New Hampshire, New York,

Tennessee, and Texas. Of these, Maryland requires that the certification be conducted by the Indoor Air Quality Association. Two states require or will require that the certification be earned through training offered by the American Council for Accredited Certification: Maryland and New Hampshire. Only Texas requires certification of all mold workers. Only New York and Texas contain exemptions in the mold remediation regulation for rental properties.[33]

Locating a Lawyer

Because of the complexities surrounding toxic mold exposure, it is best to find an experienced personal injury attorney familiar with mold litigation. This, of course, is a difficult challenge given the lack of federal guidelines. Nolo.com offers a helpful lawyer directory with a state-by-state search feature providing information about the attorney's philosophy, fees, and experience.[34]

Always weigh your options carefully when pursuing legal action. The lack of government regulation can make this an uphill battle. However, resources like these can help as you determine your wisest course of action.

Chapter 10

Your Next Home

What are some guidelines I can follow for buying or renting a home?

What should you look for when buying or renting a home? How can you choose a safe environment and avoid hazardous water damage that can lead to serious health issues?

The following suggestions are based in part on the book *The Homeowner's Guide to Mold* by Michael Pugliese.[35]

1. Look for a low permeability rating (minimal chance of unwanted moisture entering the home). The building lot should have a high enough water table and be away from underground springs. The slope of the land is a key factor to avoid water running toward the house.

2. Check crawl spaces to make sure there is no moisture. Crawl spaces tend to be damp and are therefore a challenge for mold avoidance.

3. Does this home have a basement? Is it finished or unfinished? If it is unfinished, make sure the dirt is dry. If it is finished, look a history of water damage. Carpeting is a potential problem. Basements require thorough inspection, as they are a common source of mold growth.

4. Check the drainage of the home. The roof should have overhangs to help carry drainage farther away from the structure. Check the flashing (a thin sheet used to prevent water intrusion). Improper flashing is a common cause of roof leaks. Ask about any history of roof leaks. Shingles at the eaves should project beyond the edge of the roof framing. Check gutters and downspouts to see that they are properly installed. After your move, consider adding inexpensive splash blocks to help carry water away from the home.

5. Be sure wood siding stops well above the ground to avoid stain and rot.

6. Make sure windows are installed right side up so the weep holes drain properly.

7. Avoid central humidification systems, if possible.

8. Check to see that drip pans for cooling coils are draining properly.

9. Check the locations of the closets. If a closet runs along an outside wall, the cold wall can meet the heated inside air and form condensation. Good quality construction will allow for proper insulation of these closets.

10. If the home appears safe and has no history of water damage, consider testing the home. An ERMI or HERTSMI mold test can rule out the presence of toxic mold. This can be done by collecting a sample of dust and submitting it to a lab for analysis. It is important to rule out the presence of *Stachybotrys* and other toxic molds. If you have experienced a prior mold exposure, look for a home with an ERMI value

of 2 or less. See Chapter 1: First Steps for more details on ERMI and HERTSMI dust testing. A thermal inspection of the home can reveal hidden moisture. Consider purchasing a thermal imaging device in advance. FLIR ONE offers a thermal imaging app as well as a mini camera for an affordable price.

Other Important Considerations

1. Be aware of chemical use in the home. For those with chemical sensitivities, it is best to avoid homes with air fresheners, recent pesticide treatments, and a history of smoking.

2. Consider the home's proximity to cell towers and power lines. There is evidence that electromagnetic radiation from cell phone towers is hazardous to health. Research is ongoing and it's hard to say how far is "far enough," but ideally the farther away you are from a cell tower the better. Websites such as AntennaSearch.com provide a searchable database for checking the location of nearby towers.

   In addition, proximity to power lines can be an issue. All homes are "close" to power lines, but the health impact decreases with distance. There are many variables with power lines, so it's something to keep in mind when searching for a safe home.

3. Does the home have a smart meter? Smart meters are increasingly linked to ill health. While a smart meter may not be avoidable, this too is something to keep in mind. Does the local utility offer an opt-out? How close is the meter to the sleeping areas of the home? Shielding is always an option, so this may or may not break your decision to purchase or rent.

For more suggestions on choosing or creating a healthy home environment, see the informative International Institute for Building-Biology & Ecology website[36] or the excellent written resource *Prescriptions for a Healthy House.*[37]

If health is an issue and you are looking to rent a home or apartment, consider adding this Health Addendum to the lease agreement:

Management releases Resident from lease agreement if Resident's health is affected by environmental factors associated with chemical sensitivity and/or mold issues.

Following these guidelines can help you avoid health issues and financial loss. Be mindful of the current residents' health and be sure to listen to your instincts. Choosing your next living environment wisely has the potential to benefit your family's health for years to come.

Chapter 11

Hope After Mold

Is there life after a serious mold exposure?

It's been more than seven years since we vacated our home. The journey has been longer than I'd hoped and filled with unanticipated twists and turns. The knowledge I've gained is one of the benefits of traveling this road. Thankfully, mold is not in the forefront of my thinking now, and while we do have some lingering issues, we are no longer consumed with our health. I do, however, remain vigilant and aware, and I am always learning.

Lessons I Have Learned

1. Take care of yourself and your family.

When we first left the home, I wanted everyone to know about mold. This drive to educate others drained me of energy. It also dictated some unwise decisions. If I had it to do over, I would spend less time trying to convince others and more time learning this ourselves. I would not spin my wheels trying to keep this from happening to others. We could have easily sold our home "as is" with full disclosure, but we were too traumatized to see that being up-front and honest about our home was enough. We lost valuable resources trying to protect others and lost momentum on our own recovery.

2. Keep moving forward.

It's easy to find yourself looking back with regret.

- If only I had known . . .
- I wish I had . . .
- I should have done . . .
- Why didn't I . . .

As much as possible, use your knowledge to propel yourself forward. Maybe your next step is to test the home. Perhaps it means tossing some books or clothes that are causing you problems. It may mean a radical step like sleeping outside. It could mean hiring a qualified remediator. It might be a diet change. Whatever moving forward looks like for you, don't drown yourself in "what ifs;" use your experience to take the next step.

3. Don't jump ahead.

When evaluating a course of action, it's easy to think too far ahead.

- If I test the home, I might have to leave it.
- If we hire a mold remediator, it might not work.
- If I spend money on this step, I might not have the money I need in the future.

The scenarios are endless. If your house is on fire, there is no time to think about the long-term implications. Unfortunately, an unhealthy building is far more complicated. As much as possible, focus only on your next step and keep yourself from becoming paralyzed by the "what if" scenarios.

4. Embrace the process.

After we left our home, I put time limits on our recovery. As a result, I felt behind schedule and sure I wasn't doing enough to get us well. The self-imposed timeline made me vulnerable to those who touted a specific remedy, supplement, or treatment. With time I learned there is no "magic pill" when it comes to the recovery process. Once I relinquished my sense of urgency, I was able to enjoy subtle changes and small victories. I gave it time, and seven years later I'm glad I did.

There are many others who have traveled this road. They too have learned that time is a critical part of the journey. I hope these excerpts of stories found on the momsAWARE website[38] will give you encouragement.

Lisa

Lisa recovered her health through mold avoidance and a variety of detox interventions.

"But what has mattered most is good, fresh, clean air."

Erik

Erik practiced extreme mold avoidance while embracing the outdoors, specifically mountain climbing.

"While not a cure, this is more effective than any remedy that I have ever seen . . . and deserves research."

Heather

Heather tossed most of her belongings and remediated her home. She lived between motels and tents for more than 10 months.

"My son started improving within four days. We knew we could not go back to that house until it was fixed."

Kelly

Kelly and her family vacated their home and took nothing with them.

"We have been detoxing, avoiding, and recovering
for four years and are getting better daily."

Ryan

Ryan, his wife, and their four children vacated their home and built a new one, with their eyes wide open this time.

"Everything is not better by any means, but we know we did
what we had to do for the sake of ourselves and our four
children. I only wish we had figured it out sooner."

Angela

Angela and her family lost their home to toxic mold. When she had a good day during those first months after leaving, Angela would write it down.

"Then I could look back on those days and see
how far I'd come. The 'good days' evolved into better days
and it gave me hope."

Wherever you are on your journey, there is hope. Hope for an improved quality of life. Hope for a day when more people will realize the connection between environment and health.

The mold journey is not an easy one. Narrow your focus and embrace the process. One day you'll find yourself on the other side, offering a word of hope to others.

Appendix A

Our Family's Story

A Timeline of Events

The following timeline chronicles our family's encounter with toxic mold, the vacating of our Colorado home, and the events of the following year.

June 2000. Chris, our eight children, and I move from a small 1,800-square-foot home in suburban Chicago to an expansive, relatively new 5,500-square-foot home in Monument, Colorado. We choose Colorado for its beauty and proximity to Chris' writing colleagues.

June 2001 through May 2007. Our ninth child, Brandon James, is born in June 2001. We begin to see some medical issues arise. Our oldest daughter develops a severe nut allergy. Our fourth daughter is diagnosed with complex partial seizure disorder. Other issues arise in the family, such as mild hearing loss, heavy menstrual bleeding, rashes, nickel allergies, swollen adenoids, and a dog with diabetes. We make no association with our home.

April 2007. Our 11-year-old son, Reagan, has a skin biopsy for a mysterious rash in the form of small bumps on his elbows and other joints. A dermatologist cannot diagnose the cause.

May 9, 2007 (the day before Mother's Day). In the process of preparing for carpets to be cleaned in our downstairs level, I notice a brown spot in the corner of our oldest daughter's room. It is located directly behind a bathroom. After uncovering the spot and cutting into the wall, we discover black mold. (We learn much later that cutting into the wall caused the spores to be released, thereby putting the family at risk.) We call a mold remediation team to diagnose and treat it. They do not wear masks and do not ventilate the contaminated air. They assure us there is no risk or danger. We believe them. (Fourteen months later I would read: "Remediators who are not wearing any face, mouth, hand, or body protection in the midst of visible mold or moldy odors are untrained and should be asked to leave. You will be hurt by their lack of training."[39])

June 26, 2007 (seven weeks after exposure). Our seven-year-old son, Colin, is diagnosed with type 1 juvenile diabetes. Research suggests a "toxic trigger" for onset. Colin slept in a room with little to no ventilation, which could explain his predisposition to diabetes (with toxic fumes in the home). His adenoids became swollen soon after moving to Colorado. One website explains, "Usually, enlargement of the gland indicates increased working of the gland, i.e. reaction towards the disease or infective agents (bacteria or viruses or fungi)." With no family history and little experience with medical issues, we are launched into a new world.

July 2007. We learn from our insurance company that slow leaks and mold are not covered.

September 11, 2007. Reagan calls from school to say his ear is ringing. I take him to a top neurotologist in Colorado Springs.

October 1, 2007. Reagan's ear ringing is debilitating. An MRI and blood work are scheduled.

November 1, 2007. Reagan wakes up dizzy. No doubt the sugar from Halloween has triggered the escalation of his illness. A few days later he is up all night with vertigo and vomiting. His last day of sixth grade will prove to be October 31.

November 6, 2007. We seek a second opinion at Children's Hospital in Denver. Because of the severity of the vertigo attacks, we are admitted to the emergency room. The senior neurologist determines there is nothing neurologically wrong. ENT doctors at the hospital are mystified.

November 10, 2007. As Reagan's violent vertigo continues, the neurotologist gives the diagnosis of Meniere's disease and performs shunt surgery. Reagan recovers well and begins vestibular rehabilitation as walking has become labored and difficult.

November 22, 2007. Reagan's vertigo returns with a vengeance. Phenergan and valium are prescribed. We are now carrying Reagan as his balance is clearly disturbed.

November 28, 2007. Reagan is admitted to the hospital for an injection of gentamicin with the hope of killing the eighth nerve on the left side. Following surgery he is admitted to the rehabilitation unit at Memorial Hospital, as he is only able to walk with the help of a walker. His balance is restored on day seven. He is perpetually dizzy and crying at night; the dizziness is extremely intense. The rehab people seem mystified that he is chronically dizzy. The rehab doctor assumes it must be psychological.

December 7, 2007. Reagan comes home from the hospital. The vertigo returns within days. He is perpetually dizzy 24 hours a day, awake until two a.m. most nights until exhaustion overtakes him. I have to hold him and sing to him until he finally falls asleep.

December 21, 2007. A second gentamicin injection is given through outpatient surgery.

December 22, 2007. Reagan's vertigo intensifies.

December 25, 2007 (Christmas Day). Reagan is terribly dizzy. He bangs his head against the couch to try to get rid of it. He's trying to cope with the lack of progress.

January 3, 2008. The neurotologist says Reagan needs tough love. I sense there is nothing more he can do.

January 2008. Our son with diabetes, now eight years old, continues to complain of headaches and blurred vision. He says he is seeing double. After complications from diabetes are ruled out, glasses are prescribed.

January 2008. I notice unusual rashes on our six-year-old son, Brandon.

January 2008. I call an environmental hygienist in Denver and talk with him at length about my children's illnesses and the mold remediation in May. He does not believe the illnesses are related to last year's exposure. He is aware only of respiratory illnesses related to mold. He says we would be wasting our money to have our air tested. He comments on the fact that the remediation team wore no masks. He calls it poor business practice and unprofessional.

February 2008. Our 10-year-old daughter, Kaitlyn,

continues to complain of headaches, double vision, and dizziness. She has difficulty riding in the car. The optometrist diagnoses her with convergence insufficiency and diplopia. I take her for three other opinions, including an ophthalmologist, who concurs with the optometrist's diagnosis. All agree she needs vision therapy, so we begin a home therapy program. She is clearly debilitated and is asking to come home after just three hours of school.

February 13, 2008. VNG (eye movement) testing for Reagan shows the left ear has recovered to almost normal caloric activity. This is amazing in light of the toxicity of the gentamicin drug. Meniere's disease appears unlikely. Reagan's hearing in the left ear returns to the level it was on September 11. The Denver neurotologist introduces the idea of migraine. I feel a need to pursue another opinion as this is a completely new idea.

March 3, 2008. Through an email to the University of Michigan, the head of the vestibular department at the Mayo Clinic hears about Reagan and calls me. He tells us that we created a separate vestibular disorder with the gentamicin and we are in truth dealing with vestibular migraine with some adult presentation. We begin Periactin and watch for trigger foods and other common migraine issues, including weather changes and light sensitivity. Reagan's vertigo begins to make sense. But we are still not linking any of this to the mold exposure in May.

March 2008. Colin complains of abdominal pain. A stomach X-ray shows that something is clearly creating a disturbance in his intestine.

March 2008. Kaitlyn worsens. We begin vision therapy in Denver in hopes that the convergence issue will resolve and her symptoms will dissipate.

March 2008. Our 17-year-old son Ryan's acne has become severe. He has experienced chronic cold/sinus congestion/ sore throat since February.

April 2008. Kaitlyn is unable to return to school. Her motion sickness and vertigo are escalating. We see a dramatic shift in her personality. She is negative and irritable. She lies on the floor many nights and says she wants to die. The vision therapist notices a major head tilt in Kaitlyn and suggests that there may be more going on than the convergence issue. He advises us to see a chiropractor.

April 2008. Colin complains of numbness in his right hand and has significant rashes on both hands. The blurry vision and headaches continue. The abdominal pain continues. He cries at night, asking if he will feel like this forever, since diabetes is forever. We see a gastrointestinal specialist. He suggests stress but agrees to do further testing. Colin leaves school early most days.

April 2008. Our six-year-old son, Brandon, complains of blurry vision and abdominal pain. His teacher sends home a note saying he appears to be urinating frequently. Brandon is diagnosed with dysfunctional voiding. A stomach X-ray shows he is constipated.

April 2008. I become extremely fatigued and develop ringing in both ears. My menstrual cycle has ceased abruptly with no warning; I assume this is due to the stress of these last 11 months. I also begin to notice some memory issues, but quickly dismiss them.

April 2008. A pediatric neurologist at Children's Hospital in Denver skeptically prescribes Topomax for Reagan's migrainous vertigo. With no family history of migraine, he expresses disbelief that a child can be dizzy 24 hours a day.

With this lack of support, I decide to pursue alternative/natural care. Reagan is suffering with each weather change. Because of this and Kaitlyn's head tilt, I consider a chiropractor with a head/neck specialty.

April 25, 2008. I reach the point of desperation and despair. Chris is doing his best to continue to pay the mounting bills. Three children are out of school completely and are not improving.

May 10, 2008 (the day before Mother's Day). Colin notices discoloration in his bedroom ceiling. Unaware of the dangers of mold exposure, we cut into the floor around the master bedroom shower area and notice a mold-like substance. Making no connection between our children's illnesses and the previous mold situation, we call the same remediation team. They begin work the same day.

May 16, 2008. I become increasingly uncomfortable with the remediation process. The workmen still wear no masks. Black mold is visible in the room where we are sleeping. The owner of a second remediation company comes to review the work. He is shocked at the fan that is recirculating contaminated air through the house. There is no ventilation and black mold is clearly exposed. We call the hygienist and schedule air sampling for the following Tuesday. We tell the remediation company to remove their equipment immediately. They assure us that our air in the affected areas is the cleanest in the house. Once again we hear from the insurance company that mold and slow leaks are not covered.

May 2008. Reagan is suffering massive nosebleeds each night.

May 2008. Chris experiences numbness in his right hand and lower arm.

May 21, 2008. After a natural treatment for detox, Colin becomes feverish and gray in color. He begins vomiting. His fever climbs to 104 degrees. He is visibly shaking. Diarrhea begins. This continues for the next four days, and there is black substance with each bowel movement. By the fifth day his abdominal pain has subsided. The numbness is gone and his vision has improved.

May 22, 2008. The hygienist calls with the results of our air samples. The lower level of the home has a reading of 120 mold spores. The count outside our house is 790. The count in the boys' room is 293,000. Of these spores, 207,000 are *Stachybotrys* and 86,000 are *Chaetomium*. The count in our master bedroom is 321,987. Of these, 250,000 are *Stachybotrys* and 71,000 are *Chaetomium*. The hygienist indicates he has never seen counts this high in either residential or commercial structures. The mold in this area of the house is significantly less than the area downstairs which was improperly remediated last year. The magnitude of last year's exposure has to be much greater.

May 22, 2008. We call for an emergency remediation. The new remediation team recommended by the hygienist contains the affected areas and seals off the rooms by midnight. They are in full protective gear. We schedule carpet steam-cleaning throughout the house, and vent disinfection for the next week. Our clothing, linens, and bedding are put in sealed bags and are later disposed of. Neither the hygienist nor the remediation team suggest vacating the house.

June 2008. Brandon's rashes diminish following the remediation. His frequent urination is improving. I learn that frequent urination can be a sign of a low MSH (melanocyte-stimulating hormone). Dr. James Schaller writes, "The most common cause of a very low MSH in my patients is exposure to biotoxins."[40]

July 2008. I begin extensive research on the subject of Toxic Black Mold Syndrome. I read on the website Mold-Help.org: "The most dangerous mold strains are: *Chaetomium* (pronounced Kay-toe-MEE-yum) and *Stachybotrys chartarum* (pronounced Stack-ee-BOT-ris Shar-TAR-um) as they have been proven to produce demylenating mycotoxins among others, meaning they can lead to autoimmune disease. Under certain growth and environmental conditions, both of these fungi release toxic, microscopic spores and several types of mycotoxins that can cause the worst symptoms which are usually irreversible such as neurological and immunological damage."[41]

July 2008. We continue taking detoxifying supplements. I read about the prescription medication cholestyramine, which has been proven to successfully bind biotoxins. I consider blood testing as outlined in *Your Guide to Mold Toxins*. But with the children improving, I decide to wait.

August 14, 2008. The children return to school. Two of the children become sick the first week with cold symptoms. This is disturbing, but I assume it is their compromised immune systems.

August 18, 2008. I obtain Colin's blood tests from May 5 and look for evidence of toxic exposure. His gliadin IgG is high: a level of 105.6. Anything higher than 55 indicates positive for anti-gliadin IgG antibodies, which can occur after indoor mold exposure.

September 18, 2008. Colin gets a palate expander due to the mouth breathing that developed from the swollen adenoids.

September 29, 2008. I study Reagan's blood tests from October 1, 2007 to search for clues to mold exposure as the cause for his hearing loss and tinnitus. (Vertigo had not set in at the time of these blood tests; they were taken four months after initial exposure.) His hemoglobin (Hgb) level was elevated at the time, as was his level of alkaline phosphatase (Alk Phos), which was 309, outside the healthy range of 37–250. In addition, his potassium level was low and his c-ANCA level was equivocal for antibodies. A re-test had been suggested by the lab but was not ordered by the neurotologist.

September 2008. Our dog Pippen seems unusually sick. His eyes are redder than they have ever been. Brandon becomes sick again with cold symptoms. I notice my tongue is black, my foot joints hurt, and three bumps have appeared on the second knuckle of my right hand. I take Ryan to the doctor for a herpes-like rash around his mouth. Brandon's rashes are back, as are Colin's hand rashes. Colin's blood sugars become elevated.

October 4, 2008. I seek the counsel of toxicologist Dr. Jack Thrasher due to recurring symptoms. He explains the seriousness of the 320,000-plus spore count and warns that mold often hides behind walls and in crawl spaces. He advises us to vacate the home. We leave on Saturday night at 8:45 p.m.

October 5, 2008. Chris and I take part in a conference call with Dr. Thrasher and leading environmental physician Dr. Michael Gray. They explain the seriousness of the spore count and the bacteria that synergize with the mold spores, creating a general contamination of the home. We throw away all remaining clothing and begin the process of creating a new, clean environment. We find a new home with landlords who allow us to live there month-to-month.

October 25, 2008. Colin's previous symptoms reappear. We wonder about recontamination of the new environment. Dr. Thrasher suggests chemical sensitivity. This commonly occurs in individuals exposed to high levels of mold; the detoxifying capability of the body is compromised, leaving it unable to cope with normal, everyday toxins such as pesticides, fragrances, carpet chemicals, etc.

October 29, 2008. Colin's symptoms intensify. He complains of headaches, numbness in his hands and feet, pain in his chest and abdomen. He writes in his journal that he is the sickest boy in the world and there will never be anyone who can help him. His hands are bloody from the rashes. I call Dr. Thrasher once again. He suggests bacteria from our contaminated house may have colonized in Colin's nasal cavities and digestive tract. An X-ray reveals a mass in his upper left nasal cavity. We intensify probiotic and immune-boosting supplements.

November 2008. Reagan continues to suffer from migraine headaches, chronic dizziness, sore throats, and nosebleeds. Ryan still struggles with his rash. Kaitlyn asks to leave school due to headaches. Brandon complains of dizziness and nausea. I am struggling with memory loss and depression as well as a compromised ability to multitask. I sense the need to seek medical help through Dr. Gray in Benson, Arizona.

December 3, 2008. We have our first appointment with Dr. Gray. UV light shows numerous fungal colonies on Colin and Reagan's bodies. He finds polyps in their nasal cavities. He explains more about the reality of our mold exposure and long-term effects. I begin to think about relocating to Arizona to have the other children seen and begin the intensive treatment protocol.

December 2008. Our three oldest daughters begin to connect their long-term symptoms with the mold exposure. All of them lived in the home at some point during and after the first remediation. Connections are made with symptoms beginning as far back as 2000. These symptoms include mood disorders, thyroid issues, anemia, memory loss, depression, inability to focus, rashes, sore throats, endometriosis, hair loss, and more.

January 2009. Five of the children and I begin intensive treatment in Arizona. Two more children join us in mid-January. All 11 of us test positive for the presence of aflatoxins.

February 1, 2009. Chris drives a U-Haul full of mattresses and radio equipment to Tucson. We move into a furnished rental home with the hope of recovering as a family. Within hours we have trouble breathing. Several of us develop rashes, and Brandon has three nosebleeds. Something is wrong with the home.

February 2, 2009. Most of us sleep outside. We hear from the home's owner that pesticides were recently used for termites. We vacate the home and flee to a nearby hotel. We begin a search for a safe home free of pesticides and mold.

February 16, 2009. We move into a tiny three-bedroom home in a remote area of Tucson. The home is new and has never been sprayed. We buy air mattresses. Seven of us sleep in one room. We begin again.

February 17, 2009. We begin the regimen of nasal sprays, supplements, diet changes, and exercise. We consider staying in Arizona for another year.

August 14, 2009. We move into a larger four-bedroom

home, determined to continue the rigorous work required to recover.

September 15, 2009. We receive mold testing results that show the new house is clear and safe for our family. We had done thorough testing upon learning of numerous plumbing/mold issues in the neighborhood.

October 4, 2009. It has been one year since we vacated our home. We reflect as a family on our progress and our remaining health issues. We look forward to using our knowledge to continue our recovery and to help others.

Appendix B

Resources

Websites:

- momsAWARE
  http://www.momsaware.org/
- Global Indoor Health Network
  http://www.globalindoorhealthnetwork.com/
- Jack Dwayne Thrasher, Ph.D.
  http://www.drthrasher.org
- Paradigm Change
  http://paradigmchange.me/
- Surviving Mold
  http://www.survivingmold.com/
- Truth About Mold
  http://www.truthaboutmold.info/
- Mold-Help
  http://www.mold-help.org/
- Environmental Illness Resource
  http://www.ei-resource.org/

Recommended Reading:

- *MOLD: The War Within* by Kurt and Lee Ann Billings
- *Surviving Mold: Life in the Era of Dangerous Buildings* by Ritchie C. Shoemaker
- *The Homeowner's Guide to Mold* by Michael Pugliese

- *Mold Warriors: Fighting America's Hidden Health Threat* by Ritchie C. Shoemaker
- *Why Isn't My Brain Working?* by Datis Kharrazian
- *When Traditional Medicine Fails: Your Guide to Mold Toxins* by Gary Rosen and James Schaller
- *Prescriptions for a Healthy House* by Paula Baker-Laporte, Erica Elliott, and John Banta

ERMI Mold Testing:

- Mycometrics
  Website: http://mycometrics.com/
  Phone: (732) 355-9018
  Email: quest@mycometrics.com
  (Offers both ERMI and HERTSMI testing, also available through the momsAWARE website.)

- EMSL Analytical
  Website: http://emsl.com/
  U.S. East Coast Phone: (800) 220-3675
  U.S. West Coast Phone: (866) 798-1089
  Canada Phone: (888) 831-0722
  Email: info@emsl.com

- EMLab P&K
  Website: https://www.emlab.com/
  Phone: (866) 871-1984

Medical Resources:

- RealTime Laboratories
  Website: http://www.realtimelab.com/
  Phone: (855) 692-6767
  Email: info@realtimelab.com

- American Academy of Environmental Medicine
  Website: https://www.aaemonline.org/
  Phone: (316) 684-5500
  Email: defox@aaemonline.org

- American Board of Environmental Medicine
  Website: http://www.americanboardofenvironmental
  medicine.org/
  Phone: (716) 833-2213

- Institute for Functional Medicine
  Website: https://www.functionalmedicine.org/
  Phone: (800) 228-0622

- Truth About Mold's List of Physicians
  Website: http://www.truthaboutmold.info/physicians

- Surviving Mold's List of Physicians
  Website: http://www.survivingmold.com/shoemaker-
  protocol/certified-physicians-shoemaker-protocol

Detoxing Support:
- Sick Buildings Yahoo Group
  http://health.groups.yahoo.com/group/sickbuildings/
- Paradigm Change
  http://paradigmchange.me/
- MCS America
  http://www.mcs-america.org/
- Global Indoor Health Network
  http://www.globalindoorhealthnetwork.com/

Legal Resources:

- Nolo.com

Instructions for Using the Rosetta Stone
for HLA DR by PCR

from *Mold Warriors* by Dr. Ritchie Shoemaker

- On a lab report, there are five categories of results. Each patient has two sets of three alleles, unless DRB1 is 1, 8, or 10. Those will only have a DQ, and no DRB 3, 4, or 5. Everyone else will have a DQ and one other allele from DRB 3, 4, or 5.

- You only use the first two numbers from each line of the report.

- If there is one entry, instead of two, the patient is homozygous for that allele.

- The categories are translated:
  - DRB1 = B1
  - DQ = DQ
  - DRB3 = 52A, 52B, or 52C
  - In DRB3, 01 is A, 02 is B, and 03 is C.
  - DRB4 = 53
  - DRB5 = 51
  - In DRB1, if the first two numbers are 03, rewrite it as 17.

- In the Rosetta Stone template, record the genotypes in two columns, one representing each parent.

Susceptibility	DRB1	DQ	DRB3	DRB4	DRB5
Multisusceptible	4	3		53	
	11/12	3	52B		
	14	5	52B		
Mold	7	2/3		53	
	13	6	52A,B,C		
	17	2	52A		
	18*	4	52A		
Chronic Lyme	15	6			51
	16	5			51
Dinoflagellates	4	7/8		53	
MARCoNS	11	7	52B		
Low MSH	1	5			

Notes

Chapter 1: First Steps

1   "7 Million Premature Deaths Annually Linked to Air Pollution," World Health Organization news release, March 25, 2014, http://www.who.int/phe/health_topics/outdoorair/databases/en/.

2   M.R. Gray and J.D. Thrasher et al., "Mixed Mold Mycotoxicosis: Immunological Changes in Humans Following Exposure in Water-Damaged Buildings," *Archives of Environmental Health* 58, 7 (July 2003): 410–20, http://www.ncbi.nlm.nih.gov/pubmed/15143854.

3   http://www.momsaware.org/online-store. momsAWARE has seen dozens of individuals and families benefit from this form of mold testing. Some have identified minor issues that were easily fixed, while others have found that more extreme measures were needed. One of our ongoing goals at momsAWARE is to provide subsidized funding for this type of testing, to help offset the cost for families undertaking this critical first step.

4   "HERTSMI-2," Surviving Mold, http://www.survivingmold.com/diagnosis/hertsmi-2.

5   An acute and chronic, systemic inflammatory response syndrome acquired following exposure to the interior environment of a water-damaged building with resident toxigenic organisms, including but not limited to fungi, bacteria, actinomycetes, and mycobacteria as well as inflammagens such as endotoxins, beta glucans, hemolysins, proteinases, mannans, and possibly spirocyclic drimanes, as well as volatile organic compounds (VOCs).

Chapter 2: Surface Mold

6   "Ability of Bleach and Other Biocide Treatments to Remove and Prevent Mold Growth on Douglas-Fir Lumber," *Forest Products Journal* 54, no. 4 (2004): 45–49.

Chapter 3: Water Intrusion

7   "Mold After a Disaster," Centers for Disease Control and Prevention, http://www.bt.cdc.gov/disasters/mold/index.asp.

8   "Industry Perspective: IICRC Storm Damage Restoration Recommendations," Institute of Inspection, Cleaning, and Restoration Certification, http://www.iicrc.org/registrants/industry-perspective/.

9   "Draft Report of Flood-Related Cleaning," Environmental Protection Agency, http://www.epa.gov/indoor-air-quality-iaq/draft-report-flood-related-cleaning.

10 "Reentering Your Flooded Home," Centers for Disease Control and Prevention, http://www.bt.cdc.gov/disasters/mold/reenter.asp.

Chapter 4: Mold Remediation

11 "A Condensed Remediation Plan for Small Microbial Particles," Surviving Mold, January 2013, http://www.survivingmold.com/docs/CondensedRemediationPlan_v2-1.pdf.

12 "Ozone Generators that are Sold as Air Cleaners: An Assessment of Effectiveness and Health Consequences," Environmental Protection Agency, http://www2.epa.gov/sites/production/files/2014-08/documents/ozone_generator.pdf.

13 http://www.wondermakers.com/.

14 J.D. Thrasher and S. Crawley, "The Biocontaminants and Complexity of Damp Indoor Spaces: More Than What Meets the Eyes," *Toxicology and Industrial Health* 25, 9–10 (Oct–Nov 2009): 583–615, http://www.ncbi.nlm.nih.gov/pubmed/19793773.

15 Ibid.

Chapter 5: Cross-Contamination

16 "The Issue of Cross-Contamination," momsAWARE, http://www.momsaware.org/mold-101/17-the-issue-of-cross-contamination.html.

17 "Environmental Health & Safety: Mold," Minnesota State University Moorhead, https://www.mnstate.edu/ehs/mold.aspx.

18 Seung-Hyun Cho et al., "Aerodynamic Characteristics and Respiratory Deposition of Fungal Fragments," *Atmospheric Environment* 39 (2005): 5463.

19 Ibid., 5454.

20 Sung-Chul Seo et al., "Size-Fractionated $(1{\to}3)$-β-D-Glucan Concentrations Aerosolized from Different Moldy Building Materials," *Science of the Total Environment* 407, no. 2 (2009): 813.

Chapter 6: Medical Testing

21 "Online VCS Screening Test," Surviving Mold,
   http://www.survivingmold.com/store1/online-screening-test.

22 https://www.directlabs.com/.

23 "Lab Orders for Physicians," Surviving Mold,
   http://www.survivingmold.com/diagnosis/lab-orders.

Chapter 7: Detoxing

24 "Forget Antibiotics, Steroids, and Medications - Starve Mold Out of
   Your Body," Dr. Joseph Mercola, Mercola.com, November 1, 2011,
   http://articles.mercola.com/sites/articles/archive/2011/11/01/recovery-
   from-toxic-mold-exposure.aspx.

25 Ezra, Dang, and Hueser, "Improvement of Attention Span and
   Reaction Time with Hyperbaric Oxygen Treatment in Patients with
   Toxic Injury Due to Mold Exposure," *European Journal of Clinical
   Microbiology & Infectious Diseases* 30, no. 1 (2011): 1–6,
   http://www.ncbi.nlm.nih.gov/pmc/articles/PMC2998645.

26 Janette Hope, "A Review of the Mechanism of Injury and Treatment
   Approaches for Illness Resulting from Exposure to Water-Damaged
   Buildings, Mold, and Mycotoxins," *Scientific World Journal*, Apr. 18,
   2013, http://www.ncbi.nlm.nih.gov/pmc/articles/PMC3654247.

27 Dr. Martin Blank, "Health Risk of Electromagnetic Fields: Research
   on the Stress Response," BioInitiative Working Group, July 2007,
   http://www.bioinitiative.org/report/wp-content/uploads/pdfs/
   sec07_2007_Evidence_for_Stress_Response.pdf.

Chapter 8: When Others Don't Understand

28 Dr. Datis Kharrazian, *Why Isn't My Brain Working?: A Revolutionary
   Understanding of Brain Decline and Effective Strategies to Recover
   Your Brain's Health* (Carlsbad, Calif.: Elephant Press, 2013), 412.

29 Dr. Lisa Nagy, "Household Mold and Marital Discord: Part 1," The
   Environmental Illness Resource website, http://www.ei-resource.org/
   expert-columns/dr-lisa-nagys-column/household-mold-and-marital-
   discord-environmental-illness-and-relationships-part-1/.

30 Ibid.

Chapter 9: Legal Recourse

31 "Who to Sue for Toxic Mold," Nolo.com, http://www.nolo.com/legal-encyclopedia/toxic-mold-who-sue-29622.html. Reprinted with permission.

32 "Mold in a Building You Rent or Lease," Nolo.com, http://www.nolo.com/legal-encyclopedia/toxic-mold-who-sue-29622-2.html. Reprinted with permission.

33 Elizabeth Glass Geltman, JD, LLM and Adam Hess, "Mold Remediation and Certification Laws," The Policy Surveillance Program: A Law Atlas Project, October 2015, http://lawatlas.org/files/upload/Mold%20Remediation%20and%20Certification%20Laws%20Essential%20Info%202015_11_11.pdf.

34 "Personal Injury Law Firms & Lawyers," Nolo.com, http://www.nolo.com/lawyers/personal-injury.

Chapter 10: Your Next Home

35 Michael Pugliese, *The Homeowner's Guide to Mold* (Kingston, Mass.: RSMeans, 2006).

36 http://hbelc.org.

37 Paula Baker-Laporte, Erica Elliott, and John Banta, *Prescriptions for a Healthy House: A Practical Guide for Architects, Builders and Homeowners* (Gabriola Island, BC: New Society Publishers, 2014).

Chapter 11: Hope After Mold

38 "How I Survived Toxic Mold," momsAWARE, http://www.momsaware.org/mold-survival-stories.html.

Appendix A: Our Family's Story

39 From the book *When Traditional Medicine Fails: Your Guide to Mold Toxins* by Gary Rosen, Ph.D. and James Schaller, M.D. (Tampa: Hope Academic Press, 2006).

40 Ibid.

41 "MOLD . . . What Is It All About?," Susan Lillard, Mold-Help, http://www.mold-help.org/index.php.

About the Author

Andrea Fabry is a former journalist, a certified Building Biology Practitioner, and the mother of nine children. She is the founder of momsAWARE, an organization designed to raise awareness about environmental issues, as well as the owner of Just So Natural Products and author of the blog *It Takes Time*. Andrea's road to awareness began in 2008 when a serious toxic mold exposure compromised her family's health. Since then she has found a great passion for the subject of healthy living, especially in understanding the connection between indoor environments and health. Andrea currently resides in Vail, Arizona, with her writer/radio host husband, Chris, and four of their children.

48798023R00054

Made in the USA
Columbia, SC
12 January 2019